THE GLYCEMIC INDEX DIET MADE EASY

Simple Strategies for Managing Blood Sugar and Improving Health

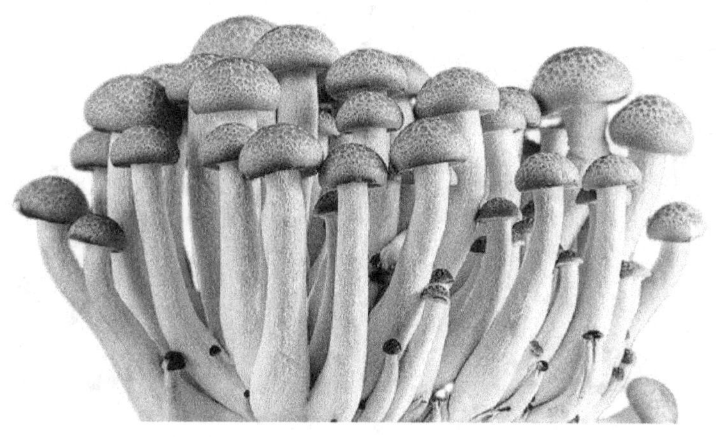

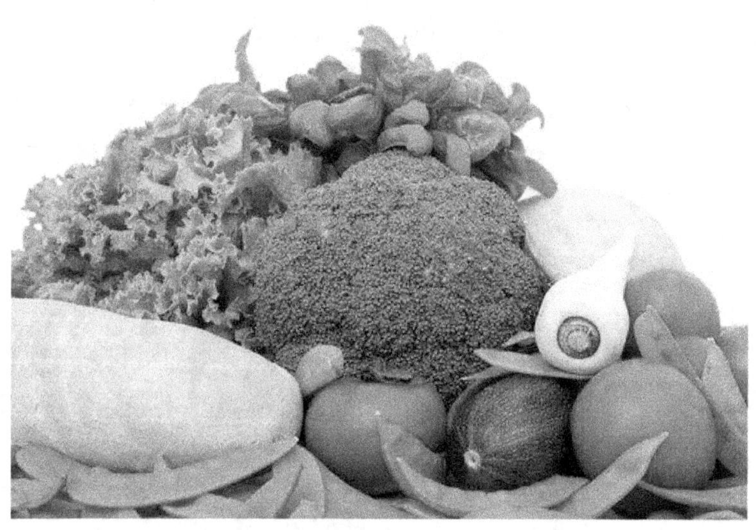

Dedication

To all those who struggle with managing their blood sugar levels and improving their health, this book is dedicated to you. May the information and strategies provided within these pages empower you to take control of your health and live your best life.

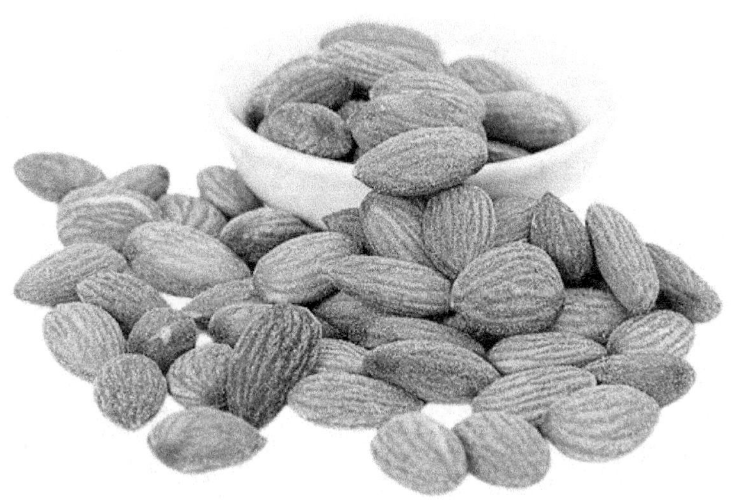

Contents

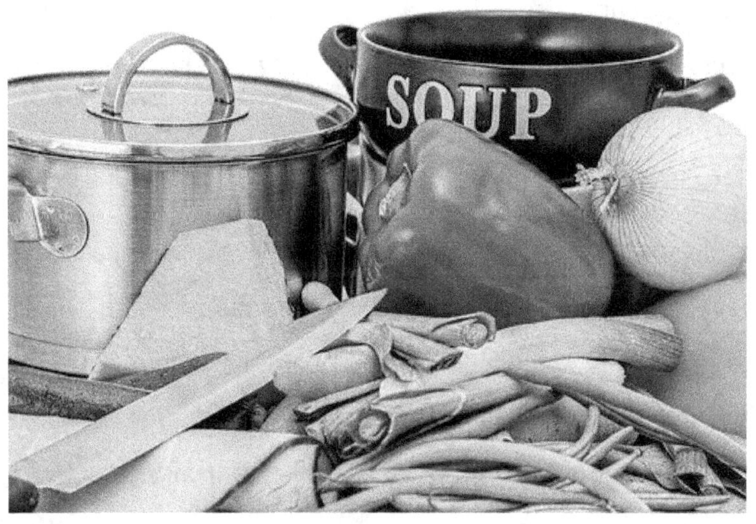

SOUP

Introduction

Once upon a time, a young woman named Sarah was struggling to manage her type 2 diabetes. She had tried many diets and approaches to healthy eating, but nothing seemed to work quite right. That was until she discovered the Glycemic Index Diet.

At first, Sarah was hesitant to try yet another diet, but she was pleasantly surprised to find that the Glycemic Index Diet was different. Unlike other fad diets that required strict calorie counting or elimination of entire food groups, the Glycemic Index Diet focused on eating foods with a lower glycemic index.

With this approach, Sarah found that she could still enjoy a wide variety of foods while also keeping her blood sugar levels in check. She was able to incorporate more whole grains, fruits, vegetables, and lean proteins into her diet, which not only helped her manage her diabetes but also gave her more energy and improved her overall health.

Inspired by her success, Sarah wanted to share the power of the Glycemic Index Diet with others who were struggling with diabetes or just looking for a healthy way to eat. That's why she wrote "The Glycemic Index Diet Made Easy" - a comprehensive guide that breaks down the science behind the diet and provides practical tips and delicious recipes for anyone looking to try it for themselves.

Whether you're new to the Glycemic Index Diet or a seasoned pro, this book will help you understand the benefits of this approach to healthy eating and give you the tools you need to make it a sustainable part of your lifestyle. So, come along with us on this journey to better health with "The Glycemic Index Diet Made Easy."

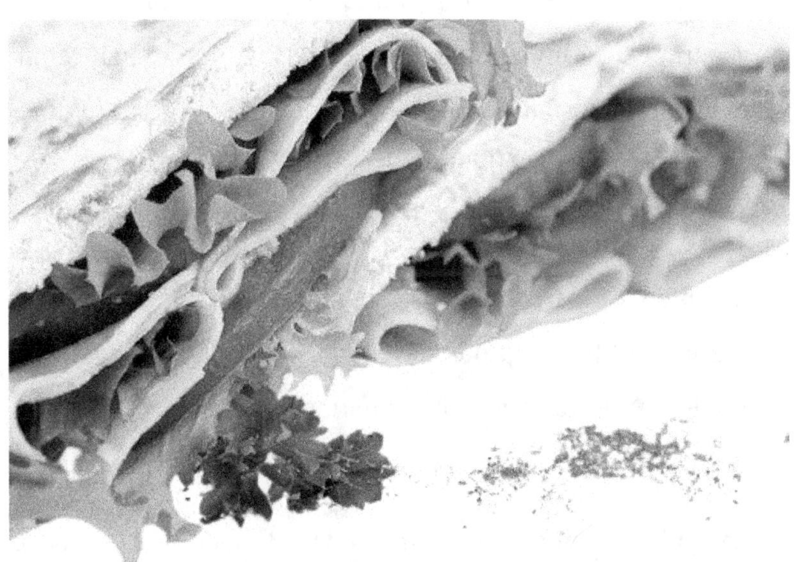

Chapter I

Understanding the Glycemic Index

Understanding the Glycemic Index is an essential part of following a low glycemic index diet. The glycemic index (GI) is a measure of how quickly a particular food raises your blood sugar levels.

Foods with a high glycemic index are quickly digested and absorbed into the bloodstream, causing a rapid spike in blood sugar levels. On the other hand, foods with a low glycemic index are digested and absorbed more slowly, resulting in a slower, more gradual increase in blood sugar levels.

The GI of a food is determined by its composition, including the type of carbohydrate, the amount of fiber, and the presence of fat and protein. Generally, carbohydrates that are more complex and contain more fiber have a lower GI, while those that are simpler and have less fiber have a higher GI.

By understanding the glycemic index of foods, you can make more informed decisions about what you eat, which can have a significant impact on your overall health. For individuals with diabetes, following a low glycemic index diet can help manage blood sugar levels and reduce the risk of complications associated with the condition.

To incorporate more low GI foods into your diet, focus on eating whole, unprocessed foods like fruits, vegetables, whole grains, legumes, nuts, and seeds. These foods are generally low on the glycemic index and provide a range of nutrients that are beneficial for your health.

It is important to note that the glycemic index is not the only factor to consider when making healthy food choices. Other factors such as nutrient density, fiber content, and overall calorie intake also play a role in maintaining a healthy diet. However, understanding the glycemic index can be particularly useful for those with diabetes, as it can help them avoid foods that can cause rapid spikes in blood sugar levels.

It is also important to keep in mind that the glycemic index is not an exact science and can vary depending on several factors, including the ripeness of fruit, the way food is cooked or processed, and how it is paired with other foods. Additionally, individual responses to foods can vary, so it's essential to monitor your blood sugar levels after eating to determine how a particular food affects you personally.

The benefits of following a low glycemic index diet are not limited to those with diabetes. Eating a diet that is low on the glycemic index has been associated with several health benefits, including weight loss, improved insulin sensitivity, and a reduced risk of heart disease and certain cancers.

A study published in the American Journal of Clinical Nutrition found that people who followed a low glycemic index diet lost more weight than those who followed a high glycemic index diet, even when both groups consumed the same number of calories. This is because foods with a low glycemic index tend to be more filling and can help you feel fuller for longer, which can reduce overall calorie intake.

Additionally, consuming a diet that is high in refined carbohydrates and sugar, which tend to have a high glycemic index, has been associated with an increased risk of heart disease and other chronic conditions. By choosing foods with a lower glycemic index, you can reduce your risk of these conditions and promote overall health and wellbeing.

Overall, understanding the glycemic index can help you make healthier food choices that can benefit your health in many ways. By incorporating more low GI foods into your diet and monitoring your blood sugar levels, you can reduce your risk of chronic conditions, promote healthy weight loss, and improve your overall health and wellbeing.

In summary, understanding the glycemic index is an important aspect of making healthy food choices and can be particularly useful for individuals with diabetes. By incorporating more low GI foods into your diet and monitoring your blood sugar levels, you can improve your health and wellbeing, one bite at a time.

In conclusion, understanding the glycemic index is a critical component of healthy eating and can help you make informed decisions about the foods you eat. By incorporating more low GI foods into your diet, you can manage your blood sugar levels, maintain a healthy weight, and improve your overall health and wellbeing.

Chapter II

The Benefits of a Low Glycemic Index Diet

A low glycemic index diet is a healthy way of eating that focuses on consuming foods with a low glycemic index. The glycemic index is a measure of how quickly a particular food raises blood sugar levels. Foods with a high glycemic index cause a rapid spike in blood sugar levels, while foods with a low glycemic index result in a slower, more gradual increase in blood sugar levels.

A low glycemic index diet has many benefits for overall health and wellbeing. One of the main benefits is that it can help regulate blood sugar levels, making it an excellent choice for individuals with diabetes. By consuming foods with a low glycemic index, individuals can avoid the spikes and crashes in blood sugar levels that can be dangerous for those with diabetes.

Another benefit of a low glycemic index diet is that it can aid in weight loss and weight management. Foods with a low glycemic index tend to be more filling and can help individuals feel full for longer periods, reducing overall calorie intake. This can result in weight loss and improved weight management.

In addition to regulating blood sugar levels and aiding in weight loss, a low glycemic index diet has also been associated with a reduced risk of chronic conditions such as heart disease, certain cancers, and digestive disorders. Consuming foods with a low glycemic index can help reduce inflammation in the body and promote overall health and wellbeing.

It is important to note that a low glycemic index diet does not necessarily mean eliminating carbohydrates entirely. Instead, it focuses on choosing the right types of carbohydrates that have a lower glycemic index, such as whole grains, fruits, vegetables, and legumes.

It's also essential to balance your meals with healthy fats and proteins, as they can further slow down the absorption of carbohydrates and provide sustained energy throughout the day. Eating a well-rounded diet with a variety of nutrient-dense foods is key to promoting overall health and wellbeing.

Furthermore, it's important to remember that the glycemic index is just one tool in making healthy food choices. Other factors, such as overall calorie intake and nutrient density, also play a crucial role in maintaining a healthy diet.

In summary, a low glycemic index diet can provide many benefits for overall health and wellbeing. By incorporating more low GI foods into your diet and balancing your meals with healthy fats and proteins, you can improve blood sugar regulation, promote weight loss, and reduce the risk of chronic conditions. Remember to focus on a well-rounded diet with a variety of nutrient-dense foods for optimal health and wellbeing.

In conclusion, a low glycemic index diet is an excellent choice for those looking to improve their overall health and wellbeing. It can help regulate blood sugar levels, aid in weight loss and weight management, and reduce the risk of chronic conditions such as heart disease and certain cancers. By incorporating more low GI foods into your diet, you can improve your health and wellbeing, one meal at a time

Chapter III

Planning Your Low GI Meals

Planning your low glycemic index (GI) meals is a crucial step in maintaining a healthy and balanced diet. A low GI diet focuses on consuming foods that have a low glycemic index, which means they are absorbed more slowly and result in a gradual rise in blood sugar levels.

To plan your low GI meals, start by choosing foods that have a low glycemic index. These include whole grains, fruits, vegetables, legumes, and nuts. Avoid processed and refined foods, which tend to have a high glycemic index.

Next, aim to balance your meals with healthy fats and protcins. These macronutrients can help slow down the absorption of carbohydrates and provide sustained energy throughout the day. Some healthy fat and protein sources include avocados, nuts, seeds, lean meats, fish, and eggs.

When planning your meals, consider incorporating a variety of low GI foods to ensure you're getting a range of nutrients. For example, you could start your day with a bowl of oatmeal topped with nuts and berries, have a salad with mixed greens, grilled chicken, and avocado for lunch, and enjoy a stir-fry with brown rice and vegetables for dinner.

It's also important to pay attention to portion sizes and avoid overeating, even with healthy foods. A diet that is high in calories, even from healthy foods, can still lead to weight gain and other health issues.

To make meal planning easier, you can try prepping your meals in advance. Cook larger portions of healthy foods, such as quinoa or roasted vegetables, and use them throughout the week in different meals. You can also make healthy snacks in advance, such as hummus with veggies or homemade trail mix.

In conclusion, planning your low GI meals is essential for maintaining a healthy and balanced diet. By choosing low GI foods, balancing your meals with healthy fats and proteins, and paying attention to portion sizes, you can improve blood sugar regulation, promote weight loss, and reduce the risk of chronic conditions. By taking the time to plan your meals, you can set yourself up for success in achieving your health goals.

Another helpful tip for planning your low GI meals is to incorporate a variety of colors on your plate. Different colored fruits and vegetables contain different nutrients, and a colorful plate can help ensure that you're getting a wide range of vitamins, minerals, and antioxidants.

In addition to choosing low GI foods, it's important to also pay attention to the cooking methods you use. Steaming, roasting, and baking are all great options for preserving the nutrients in your foods and avoiding the use of excess fats and oils.

Lastly, don't forget to stay hydrated by drinking plenty of water throughout the day. Water can help regulate blood sugar levels and promote a feeling of fullness, which can help prevent overeating.

Overall, planning your low GI meals can take some time and effort, but it's worth it for the many health benefits it can provide. By choosing low GI foods, balancing your meals with healthy fats and proteins, incorporating a variety of colors on your plate, using healthy cooking methods, and staying hydrated, you can promote optimal health and wellbeing.

Chapter IV

Low GI Breakfast Ideas

Breakfast is an essential meal of the day, and it's a great opportunity to start your day off with a low glycemic index (GI) meal that will provide sustained energy and keep you feeling full throughout the morning.

Here are some low GI breakfast ideas to get you started:

Oatmeal with Nuts and Berries

Steel-cut or rolled oats are a great low GI breakfast option. Top your oatmeal with some chopped nuts, such as almonds or walnuts, and some fresh or frozen berries for added flavor and nutrition.

Greek Yogurt with Fruit and Granola

Greek yogurt is a high-protein, low GI option for breakfast. Add some sliced fruit, such as banana or berries, and a sprinkle of low-sugar granola for added crunch.

Avocado Toast wth Egg

Toast a slice of whole-grain bread and top it with mashed avocado, a sprinkle of salt and pepper, and a fried or poached egg for a protein boost.

Smoothie Bowl

Blend together a mix of frozen fruits, such as berries and banana, with some Greek yogurt and a splash of almond milk. Top with some sliced fruit, nuts, and seeds for added texture and nutrition.

Veggie Omelette

Whisk together some eggs with chopped veggies, such as spinach, bell peppers, and onion, and cook in a non-stick pan for a low GI, protein-packed breakfast.

Chia Seed Pudding

Mix together some chia seeds with almond milk, vanilla extract, and a touch of honey. Let it sit overnight in the fridge, and in the morning, top with fresh fruit and nuts for added crunch.

There are many delicious and nutritious low GI breakfast options to choose from. By incorporating whole grains, fruits, vegetables, nuts, seeds, and protein sources into your breakfast meals, you can set yourself up for a healthy and energized start to the day.

It's important to note that not all breakfast foods are created equal when it comes to their glycemic index. Foods that are high in refined sugars and carbohydrates, such as sugary cereals and pastries, can cause a spike in blood sugar levels and leave you feeling hungry soon after eating. Choosing low GI breakfast options can help prevent these blood sugar fluctuations and keep you feeling satisfied until your next meal.

When planning your low GI breakfasts, it's also a good idea to pair your carbohydrates with some healthy fats and proteins. This can help slow down the digestion and absorption of the carbohydrates, which can further help regulate blood sugar levels and keep you feeling full. For example, you can add some nut butter to your toast or sprinkle some seeds on your smoothie bowl.

Overall, incorporating low GI breakfasts into your morning routine can be a simple and effective way to support your overall health and wellbeing. By choosing whole, nutrient-dense foods and balancing your carbohydrates with healthy fats and proteins, you can set yourself up for a successful and energized day.

Another way to add variety to your low GI breakfast routine is to try different grains and alternatives to traditional bread. For example, you can try making a breakfast quinoa bowl by cooking quinoa in almond milk and topping it with fruits, nuts, and honey. You can also experiment with different types of bread, such as sprouted grain bread or gluten-free options like almond flour bread.

Additionally, you can make ahead breakfast options that are low GI, such as egg muffins with vegetables or overnight oats. These options can save time in the morning and ensure that you have a healthy breakfast ready to go.

Lastly, it's important to listen to your body and adjust your breakfast routine as needed. Everyone's body reacts differently to different foods, so it's important to pay attention to how you feel after eating certain meals. If you find that you're still feeling hungry after a low GI breakfast, you may need to add more protein or healthy fats to your meal.

In summary, incorporating low GI breakfasts into your routine can be a simple and effective way to support your health and wellbeing. By choosing nutrient-dense foods, balancing your carbohydrates with healthy fats and proteins, and experimenting with different options, you can create a sustainable breakfast routine that works for you.

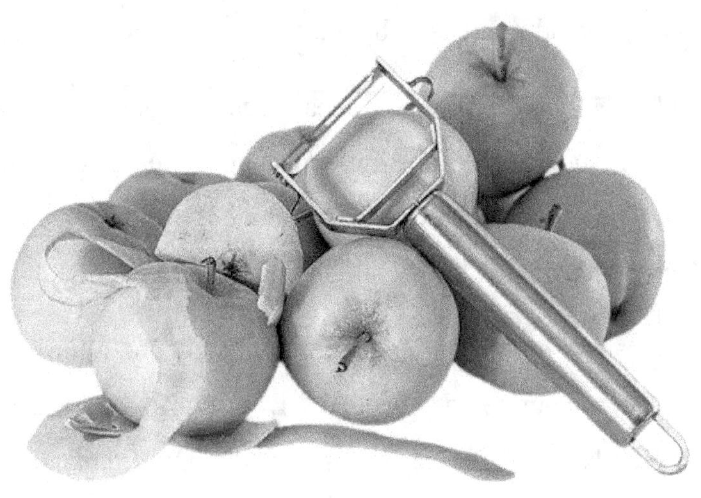

Chapter V

Low GI Lunch and Dinner Ideas

In addition to low GI breakfast ideas, there are plenty of delicious and nutritious options for low GI lunches and dinners.

Here are some ideas to help you plan your meals:

1. Grilled chicken with roasted vegetables: Marinate a chicken breast in a low GI marinade, such as olive oil and lemon juice, and grill it until cooked through. Serve it with a side of roasted vegetables, such as broccoli, carrots, and cauliflower.

2. Lentil soup with whole grain bread: Lentils are a great low GI source of protein and fiber. Make a batch of lentil soup with vegetables and spices, and serve it with a slice of whole grain bread.

3. Grilled fish with quinoa salad: Grilled fish is a lean source of protein that pairs well with a low GI grain like quinoa. Serve the fish with a side of quinoa salad with chopped veggies and a vinaigrette dressing.

4. Turkey and avocado wrap: Use a whole grain wrap to make a low GI lunch by filling it with sliced turkey, mashed avocado, and veggies like lettuce, tomato, and cucumber.

5. Chickpea and vegetable stir-fry: Chickpeas are another great low GI source of protein and fiber. Stir-fry them with your favorite vegetables, like bell peppers, onion, and zucchini, and serve over brown rice or quinoa.

6. Zucchini noodles with turkey meatballs: Replace traditional pasta with zucchini noodles for a low GI option. Top the noodles with homemade turkey meatballs and tomato sauce for a satisfying meal.

7. Grilled tofu with roasted sweet potato: Tofu is a low GI source of plant-based protein that can be grilled and served with roasted sweet potato for a satisfying meal. Add a side of steamed green beans or broccoli for extra nutrients.

8. Roasted salmon with cauliflower rice: Roast a salmon fillet with lemon and herbs and serve it with a side of cauliflower rice. Top the rice with chopped

veggies like carrots and celery for extra fiber and crunch.

9. Spinach and mushroom omelette with whole grain toast: Whip up a low GI omelette by filling it with sautéed spinach and mushrooms. Serve it with a slice of whole grain toast and a side of fresh fruit.

10. Quinoa and black bean salad: Combine cooked quinoa with black beans, corn, diced bell peppers, and a vinaigrette dressing for a low GI salad that's packed with protein and fiber.

11. Beef and vegetable stir-fry: Stir-fry lean beef with a variety of vegetables, like bok choy, snow peas, and bell peppers, and serve it over brown rice or quinoa.

12. Grilled portobello mushroom burger: Replace a traditional beef burger with a grilled portobello mushroom for a low GI option. Serve it on a whole grain bun with avocado, lettuce, and tomato for a satisfying meal.

By incorporating these low GI lunch and dinner ideas into your meal plan, you can create a balanced and nutritious diet that supports your health and wellbeing. Don't be afraid to experiment with different recipes and ingredients to find what works best for you.

It's important to remember that a low GI diet isn't just about avoiding high GI foods. It's also about incorporating plenty of nutrient-dense, whole foods into your meals. By including a variety of vegetables, lean proteins, and healthy fats, you can create satisfying, low GI meals that support your overall health and wellbeing.

In conclusion, there are many delicious and nutritious low GI lunch and dinner options to choose from. By planning ahead and incorporating a variety of whole foods into your meals, you can create satisfying and healthy meals that support your goals.

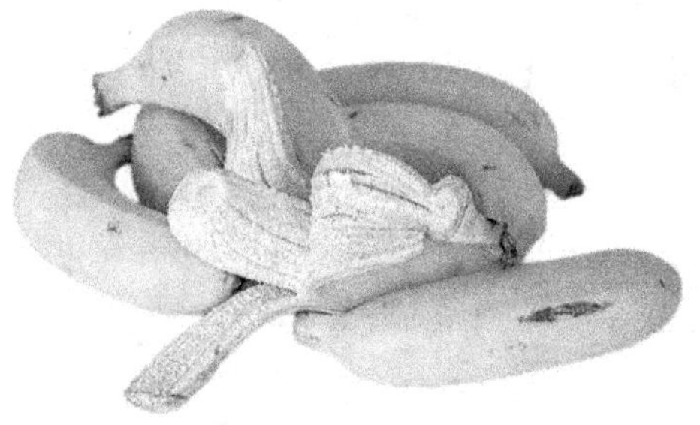

Chapter VI

Snacking the Low GI Way

Snacking is an important part of any healthy diet, but it can be challenging to find low GI options that are both satisfying and nutritious. Here are some ideas for snacking the low GI way:

1. Nuts and seeds: Nuts and seeds are a great source of healthy fats and protein, making them a filling and low GI snack. Almonds, walnuts, and sunflower seeds are all good options.

2. Fresh fruit: Most fresh fruits are low GI, making them a great snack option. Apples, berries, and oranges are all good choices. Pair them with a small handful of nuts or seeds for extra protein and fiber.

3. Greek yogurt: Greek yogurt is a low GI source of protein and calcium. Add fresh fruit and a drizzle of honey for a satisfying snack.

4. Roasted chickpeas: Chickpeas are a low GI source of protein and fiber that can be roasted with spices like paprika and garlic for a crunchy snack.

5. Hummus and veggies: Hummus is a low GI dip that pairs well with crunchy vegetables like carrots, celery, and bell peppers.

6. Hard-boiled eggs: Hard-boiled eggs are a low GI source of protein that can be eaten on their own or sliced and added to a salad.

7. Dark chocolate: Dark chocolate is a low GI snack that's high in antioxidants and flavonoids. Look for chocolate with at least 70% cocoa solids.

8. Low GI energy bars: Look for energy bars that are specifically labeled as low GI. These bars are often made with whole grains, nuts, and seeds, and are a convenient snack option for on-the-go.

9. Edamame: Edamame, or boiled soybeans, are a low GI snack that's high in protein and fiber. They can be seasoned with salt or other spices for added flavor.

10. Cottage cheese and fruit: Cottage cheese is a low GI source of protein that can be paired with fresh fruit for a satisfying snack. Try topping cottage cheese with sliced peaches or berries.

11. Popcorn: Popcorn is a low GI snack that's high in fiber. Look for air-popped popcorn without added salt or butter for a healthy snack option.

12. Roasted vegetables: Roasting vegetables like sweet potatoes, carrots, and cauliflower is a great way to bring out their natural sweetness and create a low GI snack that's packed with nutrients.

13. Whole grain crackers and cheese: Whole grain crackers are a low GI snack that can be paired with a small amount of cheese for added protein and flavor.

14. Smoothies: Smoothies made with low GI fruits like berries and cherries, along with protein-rich ingredients like Greek yogurt or nut butter, can make for a satisfying and nutritious snack.

By incorporating these low GI snack ideas into your daily routine, you can stay full and satisfied between meals while supporting your health and wellbeing. Remember to pay attention to portion sizes and choose snacks that are high in protein and fiber to help you stay energized throughout the day.

It's important to remember that even low GI snacks should be eaten in moderation, as portion control is key to maintaining a healthy diet. By choosing snacks that are high in protein and fiber, you can stay full and satisfied between meals while supporting your overall health and wellbeing.

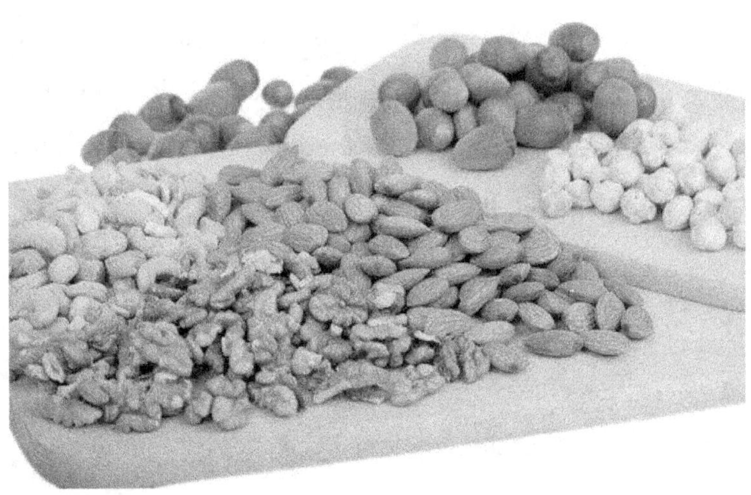

Chapter VII

Navigating High GI Foods

Navigating high GI foods can be a challenge for those following a low GI diet, but it's not impossible.

Here are some tips for managing high GI foods

1. Portion control: One of the most important things to keep in mind when eating high GI foods is portion control. Smaller portions can help prevent blood sugar spikes and keep you feeling full and satisfied.

2. Pair high GI foods with low GI foods: Pairing high GI foods with low GI foods can help slow down the absorption of glucose into the bloodstream. For example, pair a high GI food like white bread with a low GI food like avocado or nut butter.

3. Choose healthier high GI options: Not all high GI foods are created equal. Choose healthier high GI options like sweet potatoes, watermelon, and carrots over less healthy options like candy and soda.

4. Eat high GI foods with protein and healthy fats: Pairing high GI foods with protein and healthy fats can help slow down the absorption of glucose into the bloodstream. For example, pair a high GI food like rice with grilled chicken and vegetables.

5. Opt for whole grains: Whole grains have a lower GI than refined grains like white bread and pasta. Choosing whole grain options can help keep blood sugar levels stable.

6. Avoid highly processed foods: Highly processed foods like candy, soda, and snack cakes have a high GI and should be avoided as much as possible.

7. Choose low GI alternatives: When possible, choose low GI alternatives to high GI foods. For example, swap white bread for whole grain bread, or white rice for brown rice.

8. Be mindful of cooking methods: The cooking method can also affect the GI of a food. For example, boiled potatoes have a higher GI than baked potatoes. Steaming, baking, and roasting are generally better

options than boiling when it comes to preserving the low GI of certain foods.

9. Consider timing of high GI foods: Timing is also important when it comes to high GI foods. Eating high GI foods after exercise can help minimize the impact on blood sugar levels. It's also a good idea to avoid high GI foods before bed, as they can interfere with sleep and promote weight gain.

10. Check food labels: When grocery shopping, check the nutrition labels of packaged foods to determine their GI value. Look for foods that are labeled as "low GI" or have a GI score of 55 or less.

11. Experiment with different ingredients and recipes: The world of low GI cooking can be exciting and full of new flavor combinations. Try experimenting with different ingredients and recipes to find what works best for you. Some low GI ingredients to consider including in your meals include legumes, whole grains, non-starchy vegetables, and fruits like berries and apples.

12. Don't forget about hydration: Staying hydrated is important for overall health and can also help regulate blood sugar levels. Opt for water, herbal tea, or low sugar drinks like coconut water instead of high GI drinks like soda or fruit juice.

13. Be consistent: Consistency is key when it comes to managing blood sugar levels. Aim to eat regular meals and snacks throughout the day, rather than skipping meals or relying on high GI snacks. This can help prevent spikes and dips in blood sugar levels.

14. Practice mindful eating: Mindful eating involves paying attention to your body's hunger and fullness cues, as well as the flavors and textures of the food you're eating. This can help prevent overeating and promote a healthy relationship with food.

By incorporating these additional tips into your low GI diet, you can continue to enjoy a wide variety of delicious and nutritious foods while supporting stable blood sugar levels and overall health.

By incorporating these tips into your daily routine, you can manage high GI foods while still enjoying a variety of delicious and healthy foods.

Remember that a balanced diet is key to overall health and wellbeing, and it's okay to enjoy high GI foods in moderation.

Remember that the goal of a low GI diet is to support stable blood sugar levels and overall health and wellbeing. While it's important to be mindful of high GI foods, it's also important to enjoy a variety of nutritious and delicious foods as part of a balanced diet.

Consult with a healthcare professional or registered dietitian to determine if a low GI diet is right for you and to receive personalized recommendations.

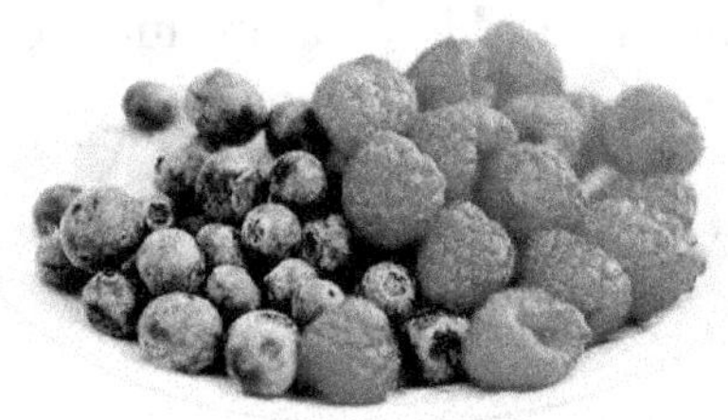

Chapter VIII

Tips for Eating Out on a Low GI Diet

Eating out can be a challenge when following a low GI diet, but with some planning and preparation, it's possible to make healthy choices that support stable blood sugar levels. Here are some tips for eating out on a low GI diet:

1. Research menus in advance: Before heading out to a restaurant, take a look at the menu online to see what options are available. Look for dishes that are based on low GI ingredients like non-starchy vegetables, legumes, and whole grains.

2. Consider the cooking method: When choosing a dish, consider how it's prepared. Grilled, baked, or roasted dishes are generally better options than fried or sautéed dishes, which may be higher in fat and therefore higher in GI.

3. Opt for protein and fiber: Foods high in protein and fiber can help slow down the absorption of carbohydrates and promote stable blood sugar levels.

Look for dishes that feature lean protein sources like fish or chicken and include plenty of non-starchy vegetables.

4. Watch portion sizes: Restaurant portions can be larger than what you would normally eat at home, so be mindful of how much you're consuming. Consider sharing a dish with a friend or taking leftovers home for another meal.

5. Be mindful of dressings and sauces: Dressings and sauces can be high in sugar and therefore high in GI. Ask for dressings and sauces on the side so you can control how much you consume.

6. Avoid high GI drinks: Stick to low GI drinks like water or unsweetened tea instead of sugary drinks like soda or juice.

7. Don't be afraid to ask questions: Don't hesitate to ask your server about the ingredients in a dish or how it's prepared. They may be able to offer suggestions or make modifications to accommodate your dietary needs.

8. Look for healthier alternatives: Many restaurants now offer healthier alternatives to traditional high GI dishes. Look for options like brown rice instead of white rice or a salad instead of fries.

9. Consider ethnic cuisine: Many ethnic cuisines like Indian, Thai, and Mexican offer a wide variety of low GI options. Look for dishes that feature whole grains, legumes, and non-starchy vegetables.

10. Plan ahead for special occasions: If you know you have a special occasion coming up, like a wedding or birthday party, plan ahead by eating a low GI meal beforehand or bringing your own low GI dish to share.

By incorporating these additional tips into your low GI diet when eating out, you can continue to enjoy dining out with friends and family while supporting stable blood sugar levels and overall health.

By following these tips, you can enjoy eating out while still adhering to a low GI diet. Remember that moderation is key and it's important to make the best choices possible with the options available to you.

Chapter IX

Sticking to Your Low GI Diet for the Long Haul

Sticking to a low GI diet can be challenging, but it's important to remember that it's a lifestyle change that can have a significant impact on your health in the long run.

Here are some tips for sticking to your low GI diet for the long haul:

1. Make gradual changes: Trying to overhaul your entire diet at once can be overwhelming. Instead, make small, gradual changes over time. For example, start by swapping out high GI foods for low GI alternatives one meal at a time.

2. Keep healthy foods on hand: Make sure to keep healthy, low GI snacks on hand at home, work, and on-the-go. This can help prevent temptation to indulge in high GI snacks.

3. Plan ahead: Planning your meals ahead of time can help you stay on track with your low GI diet. Make a

grocery list and prep your meals in advance so that you always have healthy options available.

4. Don't skip meals: Skipping meals can lead to overeating later in the day and can also disrupt blood sugar levels. Make sure to eat regular meals and snacks throughout the day to keep your blood sugar levels stable.

5. Find support: Join a support group or seek support from friends and family who are also following a low GI diet. Having a support system can help keep you motivated and accountable.

6. Be patient: Changing your diet takes time and patience. Don't get discouraged if you slip up or have setbacks. Focus on progress, not perfection, and celebrate small victories along the way.

By following these tips and staying committed to your low GI diet, you can achieve long-term success in managing your blood sugar levels and overall health.

Chapter X

Recipes for Low GI Eating

Following a low glycemic index (GI) diet doesn't mean sacrificing flavor or variety in your meals. In fact, there are many delicious and nutritious recipes that incorporate low GI foods.

Here are Some Recipe Ideas for Low GI Eating:

1. Breakfast: Start your day off with a low GI breakfast, such as oatmeal with nuts and berries or a veggie omelette with whole grain toast. You can also try a breakfast smoothie made with low GI fruits like berries and cherries, along with Greek yogurt and almond milk.

2. Lunch: For a low GI lunch, try a quinoa salad with roasted veggies and grilled chicken or a veggie wrap with hummus, avocado, and sprouts. You can also make a low GI soup, such as lentil soup or butternut squash soup.

3. Dinner: There are many low GI dinner options, such as roasted salmon with asparagus and sweet potato or grilled chicken with a side of roasted brussels sprouts and quinoa. You can also make a stir-fry with low GI veggies like bell peppers, broccoli, and snap peas, along with lean protein like chicken or tofu.

4. Snacks: For low GI snacks, try apple slices with almond butter, carrot sticks with hummus, or roasted chickpeas. You can also make your own trail mix with nuts, seeds, and dried fruit.

5. Desserts: You don't have to give up desserts on a low GI diet. Try a fruit salad with low GI fruits like strawberries, blueberries, and raspberries, or a low GI dessert like chia seed pudding with almond milk and fresh fruit.

6. Baked sweet potato: Sweet potatoes have a low GI and are rich in fiber and vitamins. Try baking a sweet potato in the oven and topping it with black beans, salsa, and avocado for a delicious and nutritious meal.

7. Lentil stew: Lentils have a low GI and are a great source of protein and fiber. Make a hearty lentil stew with veggies like carrots, celery, and onion, along with spices like cumin and turmeric.

8. Brown rice stir-fry: Brown rice has a lower GI than white rice and is a good source of fiber and nutrients. Make a stir-fry with brown rice, veggies like broccoli and peppers, and a lean protein like shrimp or tofu.

9. Cauliflower pizza crust: Cauliflower has a low GI and can be used as a healthy alternative to traditional pizza crust. Make a cauliflower crust pizza with low GI toppings like spinach, mushrooms, and chicken.

10. Greek yogurt parfait: Greek yogurt has a low GI and is a good source of protein and calcium. Make a parfait with Greek yogurt, low GI fruits like berries and pomegranate seeds, and a sprinkle of nuts or granola.

Remember, when cooking with low GI foods, it's important to be mindful of the cooking method and seasoning used. Choose healthy cooking methods like baking, roasting, and grilling, and use herbs and spices for flavor instead of high-sugar sauces and dressings.

Incorporating low GI recipes into your meal planning can help support stable blood sugar levels, promote satiety, and provide a wide variety of delicious and nutritious meals.

When planning your low GI meals, be sure to focus on whole, unprocessed foods that are rich in fiber, protein, and healthy fats. This will help keep you feeling full and satisfied while supporting stable blood sugar levels.

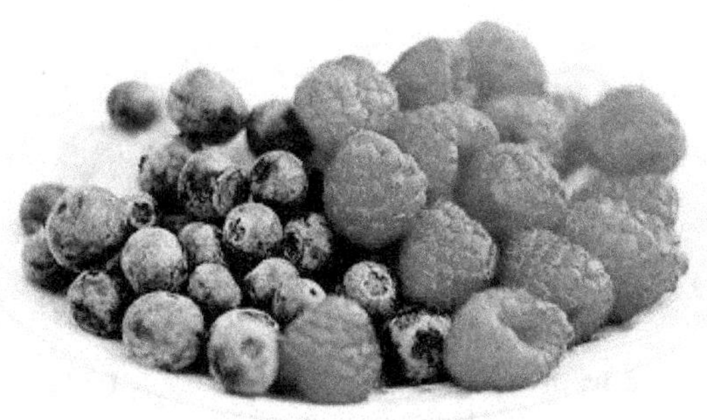

Conclusion

The glycemic index diet can be a helpful tool for those looking to manage their blood sugar levels and improve overall health. By incorporating more low GI foods into your meals and being mindful of high GI foods, you can support stable blood sugar levels, promote satiety, and reduce the risk of chronic health conditions like diabetes and heart disease.

With a little planning and creativity, following a low GI diet can be easy and enjoyable. From delicious low GI breakfast ideas to satisfying low GI dinner recipes, there are endless possibilities for creating nutritious and flavorful meals that support your health goals.

Remember, it's important to listen to your body and work with a healthcare provider or registered dietitian to create a personalized nutrition plan that works best for you. By making small changes and building healthy habits over time, you can reap the benefits of a low GI diet for years to come.